STICK **TO THICK**

(WOMEN'S VERSION)

A COMPLETE WEIGHT GAIN PLAN
FOR UNDERWEIGHT WOMEN

RACHELLE K. SANDERS

DISCLAIMER

The information contained in this book is for general information purposes only. The author makes no representations or warranties of any kind, express or implied, about the completeness, accuracy, reliability, suitability, or availability with respect to the book or the information, products, services, or related graphics contained in the book for any purpose. Any reliance you place on such information is therefore strictly at your own risk. In no event will the author be liable for any loss or damage including without limitation, indirect or consequential loss or damage, or any loss or damage whatsoever arising from loss of data or profits arising out of, or in connection with, the use of this book.

COPYRIGHT

TABLE OF CONTENTS

INTRODUCTION

In regard to what a person's ideal weight should be, a lot of emphasis has been placed on being overweight. Obviously because obesity is fast becoming a global menace. This has left its counterpart on the other hand—being underweight—to gain less traction. In the real sense of it, being underweight need to be corrected as much as obesity needs to be watched because it does come with its own health hazards.

There is no doubt in the fact that putting on extra healthy weight—for those who weigh lesser than ideal—is as difficult as trying to lose weight for those who are overweight. Maintaining a healthy, ideal weight, which in turn gives you your perfect body shape is essential for a healthy, long life.

If you are among the category of skinny people who have been struggling to add some extra pounds, you have laid your hand on a tressure that will help you achieve your goal with minimal effort.

This book is divided into two parts. The first part discusses the basics of body weights. This is necessary to help you understand the dynamics of weight gain. In this first section, you will learn how to know if you are really underweight and needs to add some extra pounds. You will also learn the health hazards involved in weighing either too low or too much. It will go further to teach you how to find out your ideal weight (this indeed is a range and not just one round number). And finally, you will learn how to intelligently beef up your weight through the selection of healthy food items and not junks and how not to go beyond the bound. So as not to land you in any further problem.

The second part will then provide you with a handful list of healthy weight gain recipes. This is going to cover the main dishes, snacks, deserts and a bonus section of high calorie smoothies.

PART I

UNDERSTANDING THE DYNAMICS OF WEIGHT GAIN

Chapter 1

HEALTH HAZARDS OF BEING UNDERWEIGHT

Weighing lesser than ideal comes with a lot of health issues. When you are underweight, it is most likely that your body system is not been well nourished. This in turn will result in a lot of abnormalities as these nutrients are needed for building healthy body cells, tissues and organs.

Being underweight is a genetic issue for some people. For many others, it is a s a result of some underlying health issues. There's really not so much to be done when the issue is genetic but that still does not stop you from been able to add a few extra healthy pounds if the right plan is been followed.

In this chapter, we are going to look at the ways in which being overweight can affect your health.

The Health Hazards of Being Underweight

We should understand beforehand that it is not every underweight person that is going to show the hazards discussed in this book. Some people will be underweight and still feel very healthy without showing any of the symptoms of being underweight.

Since being underweight is an outright sign of the lack of adequate nutrient, malnutrition is the single most important factor to be considered in every underweight person. Not getting enough nutrient from food is dangerous to health and in poses a combination of two or more of the following health problems.

Vitamin and Mineral Deficiencies

Vitamins and minerals are important nutrients required by the human body for its proper functioning. It is common for underweight people not to get adequate food nutrients and energy required to maintain a healthy weight. This implies that an underweight individual will most probably not be getting adequate supply of vitamins and minerals.

The journal, Nutrients, in 2017 published a report claiming that people who are underweight are more prone to vitamin deficiencies. When these nutrients (vitamins and minerals) are not available to the body in adequate quantities, the body's function is adversely affected.

For instances, the lack of adequate quantities of iron, vitamin B12 or folate will result in anemia; the lack of adequate vitamin A will result in night blindness; and the lack of enough vitamin C will cause wounds to heal poorly.

Osteoporosis

Based on the outcome of a study carried out in the year 2016, an underweight woman is at a higher risk of osteoporosis. Osteoporosis is grave disease of the bone that causes the bone to be porous, brittle and highly susceptible to fractures. Though, osteoporosis is a disease that can be developed by anyone, the lack of certain food nutrients increases the risk. Calcium and vitamin D are involved in cases of osteoporosis as they are both essential for building and maintaining bone mass. It has been found that most underweight individuals do not get enough of vitamin D from their diet.

Problems with Skin. Hair and Teeth

Not getting adequate nutrients from your diet might result into the occurrence of physical abnormalities in some of the body tissues such as drying, scaling and thinning of the skin, loss of hair, and dental issues.

Decreased Immunity

The immune system is your body's first defense mechanism against diseases and infections. The performance of the immune system is dependent on the availability of adequate amounts of nutrients within the body system. So, if you are underweight for not eating well enough, you are most likely going to be deficient in the essential nutrients needed for the proper functioning of your immune system. This will in turn make you readily catch infections that get in the way of your immunity.

Frequently Falling Sick

Not getting enough energy—which is important for maintaining a healthy weight—from your diet is an indication that you are also not getting enough nutrients which are essential for fighting off infections as discussed above. As a result of this, underweight people may fall sick every now and then. Moreover, common illnesses, such as cold, will take longer time to cure than usual.

Regular Fatigue

The energy we derive from food is measured in calories. Not getting enough calories from your diet implies that your body system will be running on energy deficit. This in turn will result into a body weight lower than the ideal and a regular feeling of tiredness.

Anemia

Underweight individuals are more prone to having blood counts lower than the ideal. This condition is known as anemia and it can result into dizziness, headaches, and fatigue.

Irregular Menstruation

Severely underweight women have been reported to have frequent irregularities in their menstrual cycle. In some other cases, the menstruation may seize entirely. In adolescent girls, being underweight might delay their first period. This in turn might result into fertility issues.

Premature Births

The International Journal of Obstetrics and Gynecology established in one of the studies it published that an underweight pregnant woman is at a higher risk of giving birth before the 37th week of gestation. This is medically referred to as pre-term labor.

Increased Risk of Mortality

The journal, BMC Public Health, published a study that links being underweight to an increased risk of mortality in comparison with people whose weights are average. The researchers involved in the study also added that being underweight can delay an individual's healing process after an accident or trauma in comparison with people of average weights.

Chapter 2

ARE YOU REALLY UNDERWEIGHT?

Before you proceed on your journey to adding some extra weight, don't you think there is the need to define what an ideal healthy weight is? I strongly feel we should so as not to be putting the wrong egg in the wrong basket.

It is a common practice among health professionals to employ certain mathematical equations, such as the body mass index (BMI), as a tool in the determination of ideal body weights.

The BMI is used to assess weight in relation to your height. What this imply is that there is are certain weights expected for people at certain corresponding heights. The BMI mainly is an estimation of how fat a person is and its estimation is ranged to determine if you are within your normal weight range, underweight range or the overweight range. It is originally designed by health professionals to determine the risks of certain diseases. Nevertheless, it is worth noting that the BMI is not designed to serve as a tool for outrightly diagnosing your degree of fatness nor is it an outright measure of your overall health.

The BMI has been regarded as a flawed measure. Despite that, it is still widely in use within the medical circle for its affordability and speed of estimation for the analysis of potential health status.

A BMI of between 18.5 and 24.9 is considered to represent a normal or healthy weight range. Anything higher than 24.9 is considered as overweight and values below 18.5 are considered underweight.

How To Measure Your Ideal Weight

There is a slight difference between the estimation of ideal body mass for males and females. Since this book is mainly aimed at women, only the method of ideal body mass estimation for females will be discussed.

This first method is a crude and conventional way used to calculate the ideal body mass. It is straightforward without any complex calculations.

To do this, the ideal weight for a 5 feet tall woman is pegged at 45.35 kg and this is taken as the base value. Then, for every inch increase or decrease in height, a value of 2.26 is added or subtracted respectfully. For an example, a 5'3" tall woman will have an ideal weight of: 45.35 kg + (2.26 * 3) kg = 52.13 kg. Similarly, for a woman who is 4'10" tall for example will have her ideal weight estimated as: 45.35 kg – (2.26 * 2) kg = 40.15 kg.

(Note that 12″ make 1′, so 4′10″ is short of 2″ from 5′)

This method was originally used by health practitioners in the estimation of drug dosage based on height and weight of the patient.

However, a 2016 medical study showed that the results gotten from the process described above have some correlations with the healthy BMI range between 18.5 and 24.9 for both men and women.

Subsequent to that, the above equation was modified to include the BMI and become more reliable. The ideal body mass is calculated using the newly modified equation thus:

Ideal Weights (in kg) = 2.2 x BMI + (3.5 x BMI) x (Height in Meters – 1.5).

The major distinction of the modified equation from the earlier one is that it gives more accurate results for people with taller heights.

How To Calculate Your Body Mass Index (BMI)

There are numerous free online tools with which you can calculate your BMI. One of such is available at http://www.calculator.net/bmi-calculator.html

But for reference purposes, I'll briefly discuss how this is manually calculated. I'll be discussing two out of the three methods of manual BMI calculation.

Method 1: With the Use of Metric Measurements

Using the metric measurements, your weight is measured in kilograms (kg) and your height is measured in meters (m) or centimeters (cm).

$$BMI = \frac{Your\ Weight}{The\ Square\ of\ Your\ Height\ (in\ meters)}$$

For example; if a person is 1.66 meters tall and weighs 70 kilograms, the BMI will be calculated as:

$$BMI = \frac{70}{1.66 \times 1.66}$$

$$BMI = \frac{70}{2.7556} = 25.4$$

If your height is measured in centimeters (cm), you can convert it to meters by dividing the value by 100. For example; if your height is 158 cm, this will be converted to meters as:

$$\frac{158}{100} = 1.58\ m$$

And the result will be inserted into the equation above.

Method 2: With the Use of Imperial Measurements

Using the imperial measurements, your weight is measured in pounds (lb) and your height is measured in inches.

Your BMI is then calculated as:

$$BMI =$$

$$\frac{\textit{Your Weight (in pounds)}}{\textit{The Square of Your Height (in inches)}} \times 703$$

For example, the BMI of a 68 inches tall person who weighs 170 pounds will be calculated as shown below.

$$BMI = \frac{170}{68 \times 68} \times 703$$

$$BMI = \frac{170}{4624} \times 703$$

$$= 0.03676 \times 703$$

You will then multiply 0.03676 by 703

Then,

$$BMI = 25.84$$

Note that the BMI does not have a unit.

What Your BMI says about You

BMI	WEIGHT RANGE
Less than 18.5	Underweight
Between 18.5 and 24.9	Ideal weight
Between 25 and 29.9	Overweight
Over 30	Obese

By comparing the value of your BMI with the content of the chart above, you could decide if you are really underweight as that is the main focus of this book.

Body Composition

Body composition is a term used to describe the percentages of the different categories of body tissues such as fat, bone, water, and muscle in the human body.

Weight and BMI have their limitations when used as indices to determine health and fitness. Measuring body composition may provide a more accurate insight to your health. The body composition we are going to be considering in this book compares how much the total body weight is contributed by lean body mass (muscles) and how much comes from body fat. The percentage that comes from body fat is used to assess health. This is referred to as *the body fat percentage.*

Chapter 3

WHY YOU CAN'T GAIN WEIGHT?

Now that you have been able to decide if you are truly underweight, we need to get things started. One important thing you must know in order to set off on your journey of gaining weight are the things that are actually stopping you from gaining weight and how to address them.

In the world we live today, more people are becoming so deliberate with how much they weigh and always aiming for ways to lose some pounds. Yet, a lot more people are upset about not being capable of gaining weight.

Not eating enough calories is generally the reason why almost all underweight people fail to gain weight. Yet, there are other conditions that can also make it difficult or literally impossible to put on some weight. To resolve the issue, you need to understand the reasons for not gaining weight and also look for a way to address them.

Reasons You Are Not Gaining Weight

Many reasons that range from your chosen lifestyle to underlying medical conditions are culprits of your lack of weight. Below are explanations on some of those reasons you are finding it difficult to gain weight.

Lifestyle

You might find it difficult gaining weight if you aren't paying attention to the amount of calories you need you should be consuming daily. Your daily life may be so busy that it keeps you from eating well in a timely fashion. Skipping meals and not consuming the right type of foods can also be among the reasons you are putting on some flesh. Also, engaging in serious physical activities without consuming enough calories will leave you with an energy deficit that will result into losing weight. Vet your lifestyle and take note of your calorie intake and the corresponding expenditure so as to be able to resolve the issue.

Hyperthyroidism

Hyperthyroidism refers to a condition in which your thyroid gland is too active and therefore produces too much of thyroxin hormone. Over secretion of this hormone (thyroxin) induces your metabolism to work more vigorously and this end up making you burn more calories than normal. You're more likely to feel empty and require eating too many times during the day. Yet, no matter how frequently you eat, your body metabolizes it snappily without affecting your overall weight.

Hyperthyroidism may also show some other symptoms which include an irregular heartbeat, anxiety, uneasiness, multiple daily bowel movements, and tremors of the fingers and hands. Your menstrual cycle may also change. Weakness of the muscles and regular tiredness are other common symptoms.

1. Diabetes

There are two types of diabetes, which are the Type 1 and Type 2 diabetes. Type- 1 diabetes is developed when the body fails to produce enough insulin to process blood sugars. Type- 2 diabetes on the other hand causes your body to resist insulin. Your body requires insulin to regulate the level of glucose–your main source of energy—in the blood. You may feel hungry all the time and responding by eating but you won't be suitable to put on weight if you have diabetes. You may have other symptoms as well, similar as fatigue, blurred vision, regularly feeling thirsty, increased appetite, and frequent urination. You may need to talk to a healthcare practitioner if you notice these symptoms.

2. Gastrointestinal Issues

Problems with the gut are serious issues stopping most seemingly healthy underweight people from gaining weight. The gut is where all the nutrients in your food are broken down and absorbed for subsequent use. A faulty gut generally implies that your body can not absorb what you eat. You might eat enough nutritious meals and still have to deal with malnutrition since your body will find it difficult to absorb the nutrients due to your gut issues. You cannot gain weight if you suffer from "malabsorption syndromes". Conditions in this category include Crohn's disease, irritable bowel syndrome, leaky gut, and celiac disease. You may some other symptoms when you have gastrointestinal problems – the list includes gas, abdominal pain, fatigue, and speedy weight loss.

3. Intense Physical Activities

Regardless of what you consume, you're in no way going to gain weight if you burn all the consumed calories through a strenuous physical activity. If you are on a job that requires that you be on your feet all the time, you're going to burn larger calories as compared to those who are not as active or lived a sedentary life. Lowering you're the intensity of your physical activities may help resolve the issue.

4. Psychological Issues

Your mental wellbeing as a lot of impact on your physical wellbeing and appearance. Being regularly stressed and depressed and not been able to manage it can lead to a change in your eating habits and subsequently affect your body weight. Too much fear and concern of how you look (body image) may develop into eating disorders. However, you should talk to your doctor or work with a counselor to ameliorate your condition, if you suppose your emotional issues are responsible for your weight problems.

5. Other Causes

You may also find it difficult to gain weight due to any of the following reasons.

You may not gain weight if:

You take prescription medications that increase your metabolism.

You have infection, cancer or neurological issues.

You are genetically thin and other people in your family are also born with a faster metabolism.

Chapter 4

TIPS TO HELP YOU GAIN WEIGHT FAST

Now that you know the possible underlying causes of your lack of flesh, I believe it will be easier for you to make plans that will help you take control of your present situation. Yet, care must be taken as far as what you consume is concerned. Consuming certain food might help you gain weight but not all the foods in this category are healthy choices. Some food might help make you bulky but not healthy because they add more fat to you body rather than flesh which might put you at some health-related risks. You might also end up consuming too much of sugar if proper care is not taken.

The following are a few tips to help you gain healthy weights.

Consume More Healthy Calories

You should consider fortifying your meals by adding ingredients that provide extra calories, proteins, and other nutrients. Your meals should also have high enough amounts of energy to cater for your daily energy requirements. For this purpose, you should include nut and seed or chopped banana toppings, cheese and other healthy side dishes in your weight gain diet. Adding fruits, nuts and whole-grain seeds to your meals might help increase your calorie intake.

Eat Nutritious Food

You should try as much as possible to avoid foods that provide you with empty calories. Let the food you consume be dense with nutrients. Consume enough proteins from your food in the form of milk, meat and oily fishes. Carbs should be sourced from minimally processed complex carbs and whole grains. Highly processed carbohydrates are in no way good for your health. So, stay away from them.

Snack With Care

To be able to gain weight, you are advised to have snacks between your meals. Meanwhile, your choice of snacks should be packed with healthy calories, proteins and fats. You should also avoid eating too much as that can prevent you from eating well during the main meal time. Some healthy options include protein bars, trail mix, protein shakes and drinks, crackers and peanut butter. For your healthy fats, try your hands on avocados and nuts.

Eat More Frequent Small Meals

Instead of consuming your meals three times daily, dividing the same amount of meal into 5 to 6 smaller meals is usually a way to help cub your appetite and increase your nutrients usage. It is a great way to spread the nutrients you are consuming so that you avoid possible overload at any point in time, which might not serve the purpose of its consumption.

Engage in Strength Training

Instead of doing aerobics which might constantly drain you of your energy source, you should consider doing strength trainings. These are the types of exercises ideal for the conversion of your consumed proteins to muscles. This will help you save calories and build healthy, lean muscles. Weightlifting and Yoga are great examples of strength training you should give a try.

Some other tips include:

- Drinking liquids between meals, not with, to allow room for nutrient dense foods

- Eating larger portions of fish, poultry, eggs, milk, yogurt, cheese and beans

- Preparing canned soups with milk, not water

The tables on the next few pages include information about healthy foods you can use to increase your protein and calorie intakes

Table 1: Foods to add extra proteins

Food to Add to yourmeals	Protein	Calories	Ways or foods to add it to
1 cup chopped or shredded chicken	35g	206	Scrambled eggs, omelets, salads, casseroles. Can be used with mostmeals
1 cup 1% milkfat cottagecheese	28g	164	Salads, vegetables, pasta, soups,casseroles, tacos, burritos, toast, fruit salad, smoothies
6 oz Greek yogurt,	17g	140	Fruit salad, smoothies, parfaits. Plain can also be used as substitute forsour cream
1 cup beans (boiled black, navy, kidney)	15g	~225	Salads, stews, soups, pastas
½ cup nonfat dry milk	12g	122	Casseroles, meatloaf, macaroni,meatballs, mashed potatoes, hotcereals Tip: Fortify your milk by adding several tablespoons of dry milk andstirring until dissolved
½ cup tofu (soy)	10g	94	Stir-fry, smoothies, salads, soups
2 tbsp peanut butter or	8g	188	Smoothies, toast, oatmeal, sauces,

soy nut butter			sandwiches
1 hardboiled egg	6g	78	Tuna, potato salad, cooked seafood, vegetables, salads, soup, rice, stir-fry
1 oz grated cheese (nonfat has higher proteincontent), or cheese chunks	7g	100	Sauces, soups, omelets, baked potatoes, salads, sandwiches, steamed vegetables

Table 2: Foods to add extra calories

Food to Add to yourmeals	Calories	Protein	Ways or foods to add it to
2 tbsp peanut butter orsoy nut butter	188	8g	Smoothies, toast, oatmeal, sauces,sandwiches
1 packet of Carnation® Instant Breakfast™ (36g)	130	5g	Milkshakes, smoothies, breakfast cereals, pudding
1 tbsp olive oil	119	0g	Salads, breads, soups, smoothies, sauces, fish, casseroles, baked goods
¼ cup sour cream	111	1g	Add to sauces, potatoes, dips, baked goods, casseroles
1 oz grated cheese (nonfat has higher proteincontent), or cheese chunks	100	7g	Sauces, soups, omelets, baked potatoes, salads, sandwiches, steamedvegetables
1/5 of an avocado	50	0g	Smoothies, salads, dips, bread,sandwiches
1 tbsp wheat germ	25	2g	Hot cereals, meat dishes, casseroles, creamed soups, smoothies

PART II

PERSONALIZING YOUR DIET

Chapter 5

DIET RULES

There are certain rules that govern successful diet plans. Not sticking to these rules ais the major reason most people fail on any type of diet. These rules are simple and straightforward yet important for the success of any diet plan.

Here is the big picture:

If you are starting on a diet and you feel uncomfortable with the eating system within the first 7 days, it is not the right diet plan for you. This is because you obviously will struggle to stay on such diet plan.

Your perfect diet plan must obey the SEE rule;

It must be S-sustainable

It must be E-Enjoyable, and

It must be E-Easy to follow.

On any diet that obeys these three rules, you have no reason not to be successful as long as the diet itself is ideal for the purpose it is designed for.

So, below is an overview of what we will be discussing in this section of the book.

- **Reaching your ideal calorie goal-** The success of your weight gain journey is dependent on your daily caloric intake. This is a determination of whether you will maintain your present weight, gain more weight or lose weight.

- **Reaching your ideal protein goal-** If you really need to bulk up, you will need to eat more proteins. Proteins are the building block for muscles. So, if you need muscles, eat more proteins. You might really accumulate more weight with lesser proteins but it will definitely be from junk foods. In addition, you'll only be getting the additions from fat, which is dangerous to your health. One important advantage of bulking up your muscle mass is that it allows you to eat more by increasing your metabolism. With that, you will be able eat more without much fat deposition. And that is the healthy way to add weight.

- **Making the right food choices-** You need to know what type of food is healthy for you. You need to fuel your system with the right type of food. Eating highly processed, low-quality foods is a sure way to suck in your look and heath. Your overall health will greatly be improved if your food choices are made up of about 80 percent or more of whole foods.

Your Diet Rules

The following are the only diet rules you will have to follow. Following the makes things really easy for you. They are divided into daily and weekly goals.

Rule No1: Your Daily Goal

1. Be within 10-20 percent deficit of your daily caloric goal

2. Always reach your daily protein goal

    Being in this deficit gives room for some flexibility in your dieting schedule. It allows you to be able to dine out, have some drinks with friends, and moderately indulge in things you might not find easy to let go.

Rule No2: Your Weekly Goal

1. Be sure that a minimum of 80 percent of your meals are compatible with your nutrition plan. In other words, reach in proteins and not overboard with calories.

2. Fewer than 20% of your meals should be food you really enjoy. This is even if they are not in line with the diet plan. This will give you some room for treats that you enjoy.

Chapter 6

HOW TO FIND YOUR IDEAL PROTEIN AND CALORIE INTAKE

We will be getting straight into this.

1. **How to Determine Your Ideal Calorie Intake**

   The first thing you will have to determine is the Total Daily Energy Expenditure (TDEE). This is an estimation of the amount of energy (calories) that your body expends on a daily basis. There are three major factors that contribute to the value of your TDEE. These include: (i) your basal metabolic rate (BMR), (ii)your level of activity and (iii) the thermal effect of food breakdown.

   Now let's examine each of these on after the other.

   i.   **Basal Metabolic Rate (BMR):** This is an estimation the total energy (calories) that your body expends in a day (24 hours) while it is at rest. In other words, this is the amount of energy just enough to keep you alive. The BMR takes a large percentage of the TDEE for most people.

ii. **Your Level of Activity:** In addition to your BMR, additional energy will be required to perform all forms of activities that you engage in—no matter how little it may be. This is basically in relation to all forms of movements. The more physical activities you engage in on a daily basis, the higher the amount of energy expended; hence, the higher your TDEE. This is affected by your choice of lifestyle and job requirements.

iii. **Thermal Effect of Food Breakdown:** Breaking down the food you eat into absorbable nutrients also require that energy if expended. Most TDEE calculators also take this into consideration in their formulae.

So, the TDEE takes the above three factors into consideration in order to determine the minimum amount of energy (calorie) you will require on a daily basis in order to stay as you are.

You can use the calculator in the link below to estimate your minimum daily intake.

https://www.forbes.com/health/body/tdee-calculator

The image below shows an example of what you'll get. After imputing your values into the necessary boxes, you will be presented with a reasonable estimate of how much calories you will require on a daily basis to maintain your present level of activity (your TDEE)

TDEE Calculator

The Total Daily Energy Expenditure (TDEE) Calculator estimates how many calories you burn per day.

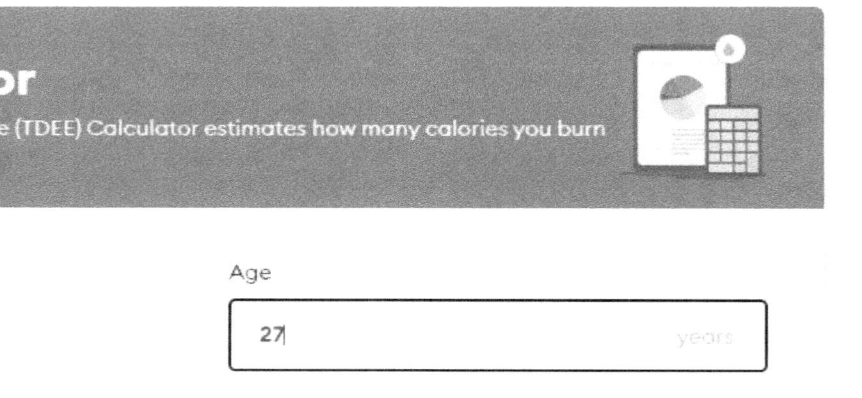

Gender

◯ Male   ◉ Female

Age

27   years

Weight

135   lbs

Height

5   ft   6   in

Weight

Lightly active (exercise 1 to 3 days a week)

Calculate >

Disclaimer: This calculator is for informational purposes only. It's not a substitute for professional medical advice, diagnosis or treatment. Calculations are based on the Mifflin-St Jeor equation, the most reliable of four commonly used formulas to estimate calorie needs, according to a review in the Journal of the American Dietetic Association.

As an example, entering the values in th fields as shown in the picture above returns the results shown in the picture below.

Lightly active (exercise 1 to 3 days a week)	1875
Moderately active (exercise 3 to 5 days a week)	2114
Active (exercise 6 to 7 days a week)	2352
Very active (hard exercise 6 to 7 days a week)	2591

So, the output indicates that for a person with those parameters and who is rarely active, a total of 1875 calories is enough to keep her at the present weight of 135 lb. For this person to be able to gain weight, she must consume in excess of the said calories (1875) daily. The excess is what will be channeled towards weight gain.

You Should Be Cautious Though

Tracking what you consume in calories might be quite easy, but it's rather difficult to track the amount of energy you expend.

So, the result of your TDEE is just a guide to make things easier and give you an idea of where to start off. What you are going to do is use the value you obtain from the calculator as a baseline for your eating for two complete weeks. You should keep your activities around this time almost the same. Take note of your weight on a daily basis (might at the beginning or end of each day but, be consistent). This will give you an idea of the correctness of the TDEE value. If your weight is nearly constant, the result you got must have been near perfect. If otherwise, you will already know whether to up your calories or augment it for your proper baseline.

2. **How To Find Your Ideal Protein Intake:** This is quite easy and straightforward. This is important because proteins are the building blocks of your muscles and other body tissues. So, a particular amount of protein must be met within your daily calories intake if you truly desire to gain healthy weights.

    Your daily protein intake is the same as your body weight in pounds but measured in grams. That means that if you weight 160 pounds, your daily protein intake will be 160g.

Chapter 7

MAKING THE RIGHT FOOD CHOICES

The secret to a successful diet plan is for it to be as simple as possible. The fewer your choices of foods, the better and easier your diet plan will become.

Below is a list of food based on categories that you should include in your menu.

A. Sources of Proteins

Chicken breast

Turkey Breast

Beef

Turkey

Lean Sirloin

Eggs

Pork Chops

Salmon

Shrimps

B. Sources of Healthy Fats

Cheese (fresh or aged)

Avocado

Nuts

Salmon

Butter (not magarine)

Nut butters

Olive oil

These should be consumed in moderation as they may take up a large number of calories.

C. Sources of Carbohydrates

Whole grain breads

Bagel

White rice

Brown rice

Sweet potatoes

Potatoes

Oatmeal

Quinoa

Granola

Beans

D. Dairy Foods

Skim Milk

1% Milk

2% Milk

Plain Greek Yogurt (Non-Fat)

Cottage Cheese (Non-Fat or Low Fat)

E. Vegetables

You can eat as much varieties of vegetables as you want. Below are my go-to vegetables:

Asparagus

Broccoli

Cauliflower

Celery

Cucumber

Salad greens

Spinach

F. Fruits

Apple

Banana

Blueberries

Grapes

Grapefruit

Mango

Orange

Pineapple

Peach

Pear

Raisins

Strawberries

Watermelon

G. Beverages

You should only consume calorie-free

beverages

Water (is life)

Coffee

Tea

H. Sugar substitutes

It is ideal that you stay off all forms of added sugar. You should even endeavor to wean off the substitute listed below. But, starting with them is a good option.

Stevia extract

Monk fruit extract

Chapter 8

DESIGNING YOUR OWN MEAL PLAN

You will have to be involved at this stage but that is the best option for you—I assure you.

This is where things get a little complicated, but I assure you that the time you spend here will be well spent.

The perfect food plan is one that both you and your goals like.

I try to avoid meal prep because it is very rigorous and provides little flexibility in your everyday eating. On the other hand, a meal plan will provide you with a plethora of options to pick from as well as a much greater understanding of food and their nutrients.

Have it in mind, at this moment, you should have an estimate of your TDEE/Maintenance calories, your daily protein intake target, and you ultimate aim, in this sense—healthy weight gain.

First Things First

Copy the chart below into a notepad, notion or work it out on a paper.

Download a calorie counting app or register at MyFitnessPal at https://myfitnesspal.com. (It is FREE)

Step 1: Make a list of the 4-5 meals you currently eat for breakfast, lunch, and dinner.

BREAKFAST

LUNCH

DINNER

> **Note:** I'll leave pages of this chart that you can just fill at the end of the book and get started.

Step 2: Ensure that each of the meal you listed above meet the following rules:

Rule No 1: Covers 20% to 30% of your total daily calorie intake

Rule No 2: Covers 20-30% of your daily protein requirements

You can use the following explanation as a guide.

Divide your daily calorie and protein goals by the number of meals you intend to eat daily (usually between 3 and 5).

As an instance:

Daily Calorie Target: 2000

Protein Target: 150 g

4 meals eaten every day

2000/4 = 500 calories each meal Protein per meal 150/4 = 37.5 grams

This does not include snacks, but it is a surefire way to meet your goals with any mix of meals you create.

- Now, enter each meal you listed in **STEP 1** into the calorie counting app of your choice and copy the meal, total calories, and total proteins into the table provided below.

You will then enter the amounts of each food in this phase. If you've never tracked calories before, this will most likely be the most difficult part for you.

To save time and for the sake of this exercise, I suggest looking for your food in the app, utilizing the default serving for every single ingredient, and guessing to the best of your ability.

BREAKFAST MEAL	CALORIES	PROTEIN

LUNCH MEAL	CALORIES	PROTEIN
	64	

DINNER MEAL	CALORIES	PROTEIN

Always remember to include the source and dressings you put on your meals for more accurate answers.

- Any of the meals that satisfy the two stated rules:
    i.   **Rule No 1:** Covers 20% to 30% of your total daily calorie intake
    ii. **Rule No 2:** Covers 20-30% of your daily protein requirements,

  Should be added to your **Meal Plan** together with the list of their ingredients as indicated in the table below.

- The meals that do not obey one or both of the above rules could be remedied by:
    i.   replacing some of the ingredients with those given in **Chapter 7**.
    ii. reduce/increase calories by removing/adding fats or carbohydrates from the original ingredients of the meal.

  Check again for their calories and protein contents and add them back to the list as soon as they fall within range.

- Do same for all the meals you outlined.

You can now go ahead and fill your meal plan as indicated below.

BREAKFAST MEAL	CALORIES	PROTEIN

LUNCH MEAL	CALORIES	PROTEIN

DINNER MEAL	CALORIES	PROTEIN

Congratulations. You just designed a meal plan that is made up of meals that you enjoy eating, and which is not strict. More importantly, you learned how to make healthy food choices.

This thus come with some advantages:

1. You have 12-15 meals to choose from, guaranteeing that you never get bored with what you eat.
2. You are already aware of the calorie and protein content of each meal on your plan. This will save you both time and effort.
3. Simply combining these meals each day will get you close to your daily calorie and protein goals.

Chapter 9:

TRACKING YOUR CALORIES OR NOT

There are varied opinions within the nutrition industry on whether you should count your calories or not.

I believe that tracking is the best approach to learn about food in the shortest period of time.

Why Should You Monitor Your Calories?

- ✓ It's the most efficient approach to learn about food in the shortest period of time.
- ✓ It's takes lesser effort to improve on something that is measured. You will know exactly how many calories and protein you are consuming.
- ✓ Breaking through an obstacle is easier.
- ✓ It adds only 5 minutes to your day.

If you wish to track, the following tools are what you'll need:

If you choose to track, tools you'll need:

- A Food Scale: You don't need anything fancy. This one is 14 dollars and will do the job just fine
- A Calorie Tracking App

I recommend MyFitnessPal.

Available via Web or smart device.

Web → https://www.myfitnesspal.com/

iPhone →
https://apps.apple.com/us/app/myfitnesspal-calorie-counter/id341232718

Android →
https://play.google.com/store/apps/details?id=com.myfitnesspal.android&hl=en_US&gl=US

Why You May Decide Not to Track Your Calories?

- You are always traveling for business
- You eat out for the majority of your meals

In conclusion,

You have an option.

I recommend counting your calories for a couple months if you want to ensure results and genuinely learn about food.

Intuitive eating (without counting calories) has a greater learning curve but may be more appealing to people who believe counting calories takes too much time.

Chapter 10

HOW TO TAKE ACTION (YOUR PATH TO SUCCESS)

You have everything you need to succeed in your quest to gain healthy weights at this stage.

- A daily calorie and protein target
- A food plan to help you get there

In general, your approach and thinking should be gradual and steady.

You don't want to gain weight too quickly. This might be unhealthy as you will gain lots of fat and less muscle. We want to gain as much muscle as possible coupled with a little fat, within the healthy range.

During bulking, you want to go slowly in order to maximize muscle growth and limit fat gain.

Gaining weight

You must be in a calorie surplus to create muscle.

During bulking you can raise your daily protein intake from 1g/day to 1-1.5g/day.

To see results, simply repeat the following cycle:

1. Meet your daily calorie and protein targets.

2. Adhere to your workout program

3. Start doing cardio or everyday exercise (I still do cardio when I'm bulking) for a few weeks until you begin to plateau (stop gaining weight). Then all you have to do is a combination of:

1. Increase your calorie intake

2. Reduce your cardio.

Then you'll have a new calorie goal to work toward, but the rest of the steps will remain the same.

This approach is repeated until your objectives are met.

For example:

An example of how this may appear in practice.

Initial Strategy

- Calorie Goal: 2000/day

- 200 grams of protein each day

- 4 times 15-minute cardio sessions each week (treadmill or jugging)

I'd do this until I stopped gaining weight/hit a plateau.

Here's how I broke through the plateau:

1. I would up my calorie intake to 2200.

2. I would not cut back on my cardio sessions.

- Calorie Goal: 2200 per day

- Protein Goal: 200g every day

- 4 times 15-minute cardio sessions each week (treadmill or jugging)

Then I'd repeat the process until I reached my target weight.

Thank You for Choosing Our Weight Gain Guide!

Dear Readers,

I want to express our heartfelt gratitude for choosing our weight gain guide to help you on your journey to achieving your health and fitness goals. I understand that weight gain can be a challenging and personal process, and we appreciate the trust you have placed in us to guide you through it.

I am committed to providing reliable and effective information to our readers. Our aim is not only to help you gain weight in a healthy and sustainable way but also to empower you with the knowledge and tools necessary for long-lasting success.

I sincerely hope that our weight gain guide has provided you with valuable insights, practical tips, and actionable strategies. Our ultimate objective is to see you achieve your desired weight and feel confident and happy in your own skin.

Your feedback is of utmost importance to me, as it allows me to continually improve and refine our guide for the benefit of future readers. I kindly request that you take a few moments to provide us with your sincere feedback. Whether it's suggestions for additional content, areas of improvement, or positive testimonials, your input will immensely help us better serve you and others seeking similar guidance.

To provide your feedback, you can leave a sincere review on this book. We truly value your opinion and want to assure you that your feedback will be taken seriously and used constructively to enhance the quality and effectiveness of our guide.

In addition, I encourage you to take action and implement the strategies outlined in our guide. Remember, true progress comes from consistent effort and dedication. We believe in your ability to succeed and are here to support you every step of the way.

Thank you once again for choosing this weight gain guide. I genuinely appreciate your trust, and I look forward to hearing about your achievements. Together, let's continue towards a healthier and happier you!

Wishing you great success on your weight gain journey!

Sincerely,

Rachelle K. Sanders

Step 1: Make a list of the 4-5 meals you currently eat for breakfast, lunch, and dinner.

BREAKFAST

BREAKFAST

BREAKFAST

Step 2: Check protein and calories contents of your meals.

BREAKFAST MEALS	CALORIES	PROTEIN

LUNCH MEALS	CALORIES	PROTEIN

DINNER MEALS	CALORIES	PROTEIN

Step 2: Your final meals for planning.

BREAKFAST MEALS	CALORIES	PROTEIN

LUNCH MEALS	CALORIES	PROTEIN

DINNER MEALS	CALORIES	PROTEIN

Introducing: "High Calories Recipes for Weight Gain"

Dear Readers,

I'm thrilled to announce the release of our latest companion book to the weight gain guide you have already embraced. Say hello to "High Calories Recipes for Weight Gain" - a comprehensive cookbook designed to amplify your progress and help you gain healthy weight faster.

I understand that achieving your weight gain goals entails more than just having the right knowledge and tips. It also involves nourishing your body with the right foods. That's why I have carefully curated over 50 delicious and nutritious recipes that are specifically designed to boost your calorie intake.

"High Calories Recipes for Weight Gain" is thoughtfully crafted with a diverse range of meals, snacks, and smoothies that are both mouthwatering and strategically formulated to provide the essential nutrients your body needs to gain weight effectively. Each recipe includes detailed preparation instructions and a comprehensive breakdown of nutritional information, giving you the power to make informed choices about what you're consuming.

Whether you're looking for hearty breakfast options, satisfying lunch and dinner ideas, or tasty snacks and smoothies to keep you going throughout the day, this cookbook is your ultimate weight gain resource.

By incorporating these high-calorie recipes into your daily routine, you can enjoy nourishing and flavorful meals while actively working towards your weight gain goals. From protein-packed entrees to nutrient-dense snacks, this cookbook offers a variety of options to cater to your preferences and dietary needs.

Remember, gaining weight in a healthy way is not just about consuming excess calories—it's about consuming the right kind of calories. With "High Calories Recipes for Weight Gain", we've taken the guesswork out of meal planning, allowing you to focus on enjoying the journey while achieving the results you desire.

You can find "High Calories Recipes for Weight Gain" on our website [website] or at your favorite online retailer. We are excited to share this invaluable resource with you and look forward to hearing about the positive impact it has on your weight gain journey.

Thank you for your continued support and trust in our mission to help you achieve your health and fitness goals. Together, let's transform your body and life with the power of delicious, high-calorie meals!

Wishing you success and satisfaction on your path to gaining weight healthily.

BONUS

21-DAY HIGH CALORIE MEAL PLAN

	BREAKFAST	LUNCH	DINNER	SNACK/DESSERT
	WEEK 1			
DAY 1	Carrot Cake Overnight Oatmeal	Chicken Shawarma Quinoa Bowl	Keto Crockpot Chicken	Yogurt Parfait
DAY 2	Croissant Breakfast Sandwich	Herb Chicken Couscous	Vegan Pulled Jackfruit Sandwich	Apple Pie à la Mode
DAY 3	Chickpea Salad	Mushroom Carnitas Bowl	Chicken Peri Peri	Veggies & Hummus
DAY 4	Vegan Protein Salad	Red Kidney Bean Burger Bowl	Chicken Thighs with Broccoli Salad	High-Protein Gelatin
DAY 5	Keto Pork Pie	Chicken Farro Salad	One Pot Cream Mushroom Chicken Pasta	Hard-Boiled Eggs
DAY 6	Baked Chicken and Rice	Chicken Avocado Salad	Beef Ragu	Instant Vanilla Pudding
DAY 7	Vegan Pesto Pasta	Sloppy Joe Casserole	Beef Stroganoff	Peanut Butter with Apple Slices

WEEK 2				
	BREAKFAST	LUNCH	DINNER	SNACK/DESSERT
DAY 8	Carrot Cake Overnight Oatmeal	Chicken Shawarma Quinoa Bowl	Crockpot Pork Chops	String Cheese with Whole-Wheat Crackers
DAY 9	Croissant Breakfast Sandwich	Herb Chicken Couscous	Salmon and Leek Risotto	Trail Mix
DAY 10	Chickpea Salad	Mushroom Carnitas Bowl	Honey Garlic Chicken	Lemon Smoothie
DAY 11	Vegan Protein Salad	Red Kidney Bean Burger Bowl	Keto Crockpot Chicken	High-Protein Milk
DAY 12	Keto Pork Pie	Chicken Farro Salad	Chicken Alfredo Bake	Cocoa Almond Shake
DAY 13	Baked Chicken and Rice	Chicken Avocado Salad	Salmon with Veggies	Peach Shake
DAY 14	Vegan Pesto Pasta	Sloppy Joe Casserole	Peri Peri Chicken	Frosty Hot Cocoa

WEEK 3

	BREAKFAST	LUNCH	DINNER	SNACK/DESSERT
DAY 15	Vegan Protein Salad	Sloppy Joe Casserole	Beef Ragu	Yogurt Parfait
DAY 16	Croissant Breakfast Sandwich	Chicken Farro Salad	Peri Peri Chicken	High-Protein Gelatin
DAY 17	Baked Chicken and Rice	Chicken Shawarma Quinoa Bowl	Vegan Pulled Jackfruit Sandwich	Cottage Cheese & Berries
DAY 18	Salmon with Veggies	Cheesy Chicken Noodle Casserole	Chicken Thighs with Broccoli Salad	Instant Vanilla Pudding
DAY 19	Keto Pork Pie	Herb Chicken Couscous	Crockpot Pork Chops	Peanut Butter with Apple Slices
DAY 20	Vegan Pesto Pasta	Mushroom Carnitas Bowl	Salmon and Leek Risotto	String Cheese with Whole-Wheat Crackers
DAY 21	Chickpea Salad	Red Kidney Bean Burger Bowl	Honey Garlic Chicken	Waffle with Toppings

I hope this 21-day meal plan using the meals and snacks provided is practical and enjoyable for you! Remember to adjust the portion sizes and ingredients to fit your personal dietary needs and preferences.